Farès Azaiez

Angioplasty of the ostium of the anterior interventricular artery

Farès Azaiez

Angioplasty of the ostium of the anterior interventricular artery

Technical approaches and medium-term results

ScienciaScripts

Cover image: www.ingimage.com

This book is a translation from the original published under ISBN 978-620-6-72471-1.

Publisher:
Sciencia Scripts
is a trademark of
Dodo Books Indian Ocean Ltd. and OmniScriptum S.R.L publishing group

120 High Road, East Finchley, London, N2 9ED, United Kingdom
Str. Armeneasca 28/1, office 1, Chisinau MD-2012, Republic of Moldova, Europe
Printed at: see last page
ISBN: 978-620-8-17727-0

TABLE OF CONTENTS

INTRODUCTION

Significant stenosis of the ostial anterior interventricular artery (AIA) is a complex lesion that poses a technical and procedural challenge for the interventional cardiologist during percutaneous coronary intervention (PCI).

Classified as a bifurcation lesion of the left common trunk (LCT) [1], it is associated with a spontaneously poor prognosis due to the extent of the myocardial territory at risk and the risk of sudden death in the event of acute occlusion [2-4].

Ostial location is also characterised by the more frequent presence of calcifications and fibrosis compared with non-ostial lesions, making it an independent risk factor for restenosis and ischaemic recurrence [5, 6].

The optimal percutaneous strategy for treating ostial stenosis of the LAI remains uncertain, according to the recent consensus document from the European Bifurcation Club (EBC) [7].

In terms of stent positioning, two basic strategies are possible: Ostial stenting (OS) from the IVA and Crossover stenting (CS) from the TCG to the IVA. Based on endocoronary imaging studies showing that ostial lesions of the IVA frequently extend to the distal TCG, it has been suggested that CS is a better angioplasty technique than OS [8].

However, data on the long-term results of these two strategies with current stents are inconclusive.

The objectives of our work were to :

1- To describe the epidemiological, clinical and angiographic characteristics of patients who have undergone ostial VIA PCI.

2- To establish the medium-term prognosis of these patients according to the PCI technique used (OS or CS).

METHODS

1 - Type of study

This was a monocentric, retrospective, descriptive study conducted in the cardiology department of Mongi Slim La Marsa Hospital over a three-year period from January 2019 to December 2021.

2 - Population studied

All patients who underwent ostial VIA PCI during the study period were retrospectively analysed.

2- 1- Inclusion criteria

- Angioplasty of the ostial IVA

- Age ≥ 18 years

2- 2- Non-inclusion criteria

- Previous coronary artery bypass surgery

- Previous ostial IVA angioplasty

2- 3- Exclusion criteria

- The presence of a TCG plaque on angiographic analysis
- Patients lost to follow-up before the end of the follow-up period

3- Methodology

3- 1- Data collection

Patients were referred from emergency departments, outpatient clinics, peripheral cardiology departments or free-lance cardiologists. They were were hospitalised and treated in the cardiology department of the Mongi Slim La Marsa hospital. For each patient, we drew up a form reporting the epidemiological, clinical and angiographic data, as well as the therapeutic and development modalities.

The data collected was :

- Socio-demographic data.
- Cardiovascular risk factors.
- Peripheral vascular involvement and other comorbidities.

- Clinical presentation.

- Angio-coronary data.

- Interventional procedural data.

- In-hospital follow-up.

- Evolution.

Creatinine clearance was calculated using the simplified MDRD (Modification of Diet in Renal Disease) formula, and chronic renal failure (CRF) was considered if clearance was ≤60 ml/min. All coronary angiograms and angioplasties were reviewed by a senior interventional cardiologist in order to specify the angiographic characteristics and calculate the SYNTAX Score based on visual assessment of the lesions.

3- 2- Angioplasty procedure

The two main techniques for PCI of the ostial VIA were :

- Focal ostial stenting of the IVA without spilling into the TCG (OS)

- Crossover stenting of the TCG in the axis of the IVA (CS)

The choice of technique was left to the operator's discretion.

The patients were divided into two groups: OS and CS.

Scheduled angioplasty procedures were usually performed using active stents, except in special situations. Angioplasties performed on an ad hoc or emergency basis used bare stents and/or active stents, depending on the availability of the latter. All patients received, before or during angioplasty, a double anti-platelet aggregation treatment based on Aspegic® (250mg intravenous loading dose) and Clopidogrel (300mg or 600mg loading dose) and/or Ticagrelor (180mg loading dose). Unfractionated heparin was administered intra-procedurally at a dose of 70 IU/Kg. The use of GPIIbIIIa inhibitors was at the discretion of the operators. Monitoring for at least 24 hours after angioplasty was recommended for all our patients. Subsequent follow-up was ensured either at our outpatient clinic, or via the corresponding doctor, and failing that, by telephone contact with the patient or his family.

3- 3- Definitions

_A stenosis of the ostial IVA is considered significant if it is ≥50%.

_Ostial location: a lesion is said to be ostial when it starts within the first three millimetres of the vessel.

_Bifurcation: this is a division o f a main branch into two vessels ≥1.5 millimetres in diameter. For lesions of the distal TCG, The Medina classification of bifurcation lesions was used to describe them.

_ Angiographic success: is defined by residual angiographic stenosis <30% at the target lesion and <50% on the daughter branch with TIMI 3 flow at the level of both vessels.

_ Procedural success: is defined by angiographic success without the occurrence of major intra-hospital cardiac events.

_ Myocardial infarction (MI): is defined according to the 3ème universal definition of MI [9].

_ Intrastent restenosis: (ISR) is defined by a stenosis ≥50% at the angioplasty site (including the stent and the 5 mm upstream and downstream).

- Target Lesion Revascularisation (TLR) [10]: Defined by any percutaneous or surgical revascularisation of the target vessel caused by an ISR or complication on the target lesion including 5 mm upstream or downstream of the stent.

- Major adverse cardiac events or MACE (Major Adverse Cardiac Events) [10]: is a combined criterion defined by the occurrence of death from any cause, MI or TLR.

- Stent thrombosis (ST): has been defined according to the Academic Research Consortium (ARC) classification [11] :

- Definite thrombosis: in the event of angiographic or autopsy confirmation of thrombosis.

- Probable thrombosis: defined as any unexplained death within the first 30 days after stent implantation or the occurrence of MDI in the area corresponding to the stent implantation without angiographic confirmation.

- Possible thrombosis: in the event of unexplained death occurring more than 30 days after stent implantation.

TS were classified according to the date of onset of thrombosis:

_Acute: within 24 hours of PCI.

_Subacute: between the second day and the 30ème day following the PCI.

_Late: between 31ème and one year after the PCI.

_Very late: more than one year after PCI.

3- 4- Judging criteria

The primary endpoint was the occurrence of **MACE** during the **1-year** follow-up period.

3- 5- Bibliographical research

The search engines used in our study were :

- PubMed (Medline)

- ScienceDirect

- ClinicalKey

- Google Scholar

- Cochrane Library

The keywords used in French were :

- Ostial anterior interventricular artery

- Angioplasty

- Stent

The keywords used in English were :

- Ostial left anterior descending artery

- Percutaneous coronary intervention

The search for these keywords on PubMed was carried out at the level of Medical Subject Headings (MeSH: keywords from the National Library of Medicine thesaurus) and Text Word (words in the text of articles).

3- 6- Data entry and analysis

The data were entered into Excel and then exported and analysed using SPSS version 23 software.

We calculated simple frequencies and relative frequencies for the qualitative variables.

We calculated means with standard deviations, medians with interquartile ranges and the range for quantitative variables.

Survival data were studied by establishing survival curves using the Kaplan Meier method.

The search for prognostic factors for survival was carried out using univariate analysis (factor by factor), after transformation of continuous variables into categorical variables according to median or risk levels in the literature, by comparing survival curves using the Log rank test.

The significance level of p was set at ≤ 0.05.

3- 7- Ethical considerations

We declare that we have had no conflicts of interest and that we have respected medical confidentiality for all cases that have been treated in our department.

RESULTS

During the study period, 1400 PCIs were performed in the catheterisation room at the Mongi Slim La Marsa Hospital. 148 patients underwent ostial VIA PCI, 50 of whom met the selection criteria (Figure 1).

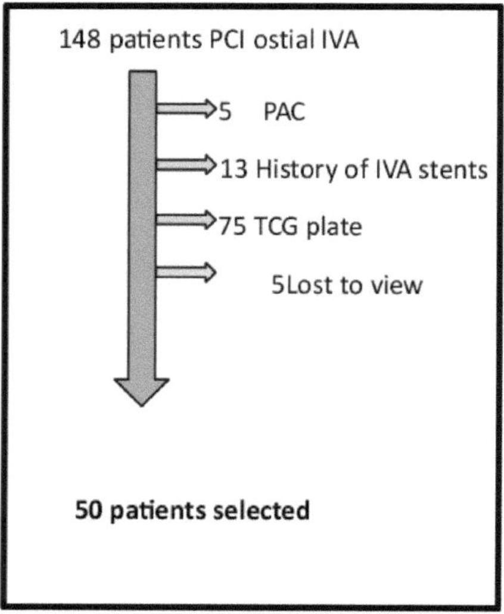

Figure 1: Flow chart showing patient selection

The patients selected were divided into **two groups** according to the ostial IVA angioplasty strategy:

- **1er group** = **OS** (focal ostial stenting of the IVA without spilling into the TCG); **23 patients**

- **2ème group** = **CS** (stenting of the TCG in the axis of the IVA); **27 patients**

1- General characteristics of the population

Our population had a mean age of 63.5 ± 14 years, with a clear male preponderance and a sex ratio of 6.14. Smoking was the predominant risk factor (94%). Two-thirds of the patients were diabetic, equally between the two groups.Twenty patients (40%) had a history of coronary angioplasty. Chronic coronary syndrome accounted for half of the clinical presentations. Only three patients (6%) were in cardiogenic shock at the time of admission.On statistical analysis, the two groups were comparable on all demographic and clinical characteristics (Table I).

Table I: Demographic and clinical characteristics of the population

	Total N = 50	Gr 1: OS N = 23	Gr 2: CS N = 27	P
Age (years)	63,5 ±14	62,7 ±13,2	64,1 ±14,4	0,67
Female (%)	7 (14)	3 (13)	4 (15)	0,73
Smoking (%)	47 (94)	21 (91)	26 (96)	0,81
Diabetes (%)	31 (62)	14 (61)	17 (63)	0,77
HTA (%)	20 (40)	9 (39)	11 (41)	0,42
Dyslipidaemia (%)	17 (34)	7 (30)	10 (37)	0,65
CRI (%)	13 (26)	7 (30)	6 (22)	0,55
HISTORY OF PCI (%)	20 (40)	10 (43)	10 (37)	0,69
CAP HISTORY (%)	0	0	0	
Clinical presentations (%) SCC Unstable angina NSTEMI STEMI	28 (56) 7 (14) 7 (14) 8 (16)	13 (57) 3 (13) 3 (13) 3 (13)	15 (55) 4 (15) 4 (15) 5 (19)	0,32 0,43 0,43 0,33
Cardiogenic shock (%)	3 (6)	1 (8)	2 (7)	0,11
LVEF (%)	50	51	49	0,23

ATCD: past history; LVEF: left ventricular ejection fraction; HTA: high blood pressure; PCI: percutaneous coronary intervention; CKD: chronic renal failure; NSTEMI: Non-ST-segment Elevation Myocardial Infarction; CABG: coronary artery bypass graft; STEMI: ST-segment Elevation Myocardial Infarction.

2- Angiographic and procedural characteristics of the population

When the stents implanted in the two groups were compared, there was a significant difference, with a smaller diameter and length of stent in the OS group. In the OS group, bare stents were used in two cases and balloon angioplasty alone (POBA) in one case (Figure 2). In the CS group, only active stents were used. The rotablator was used in only one case, and this was in the CS group. Procedural success was achieved in 49 procedures (98%). Fluoroscopy time did not differ significantly between procedures, but the amount of iodinated contrast medium (ICP) was significantly higher in the OS group.

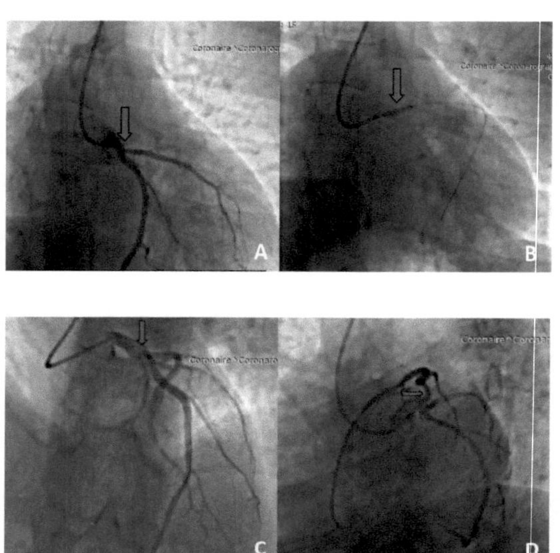

Figure 2: Balloon angioplasty of the ostial IVA in a 31-year-old man admitted for previous MI. A: Acute occlusion of the ostial AVI (arrow). B: Balloon angioplasty (arrow). C and D: Recanalisation of the ostial IVA without stent (arrow).

All the angiographic and procedural characteristics are summarised in Table II.

Table II: Angiographic and procedural characteristics of the population

	Group 1: OS N = 23	Group 2: CS N = 27	P
Stent diameter (mm)	3,1 ± 0,3	3,4 ± 0,4	< 0,001
Stent length (mm)	14,3 ± 3,2	25,6 ± 4,2	< 0,001
Number of stents	1,51 ±0,8	1,54 ±0,74	0,21
BMS (%) DES (%) POBA (%)	2 20 (87) 1	0 27 (100) 0	0,07
Thromboaspiration (%)	3 (13)	2 (7)	0,14
Rotablator (%)	0	1 (4)	0,3
Procedural success (%)	22 (96)	27 (100)	0,65
Pinching of the Cx >50%. (%)	3 (13)	10 (37)	< 0,001
Secondary Cx angioplasty (%)	0	2 (7)	< 0,001
Kissing Balloon (%)	0	1 (4)	0,3
Time of fluoroscopy (min)	10,4 ±4,4	9,6 ±3,1	0,09
Contrast medium (mL)	100 ±10	85 ±8	< 0,001

BMS: bare-metal stent; Cx: circumflex artery; DES: drug-eluting stent; POBA: plain old balloon angioplasty

3- One-year results

Over a one-year follow-up of all patients in both groups, there was a very low rate of MACE in 3 and 4 patients respectively (13% vs 15%, p=0.11). Only one case of SV was noted. This was a 45-year-old patient who had undergone ostial IVA stenting 10 days previously. She underwent recanalisation of the IVA by balloon and thromboaspiration with a good result (Figure 3).

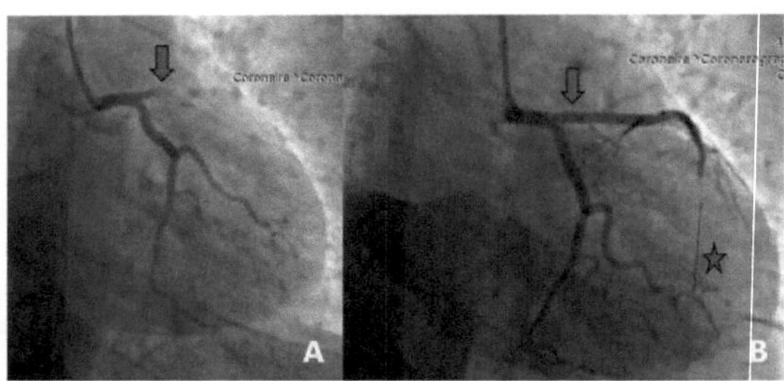

Figure 3: A case of ostial IVA stent thrombosis. A: Subacute stent thrombosis (arrow). B: Repermeabilisation of the IVA (arrow) with distal embolisation of the thrombus (star).

At the end of follow-up, only one patient died in the CS group, while none died in the OS group (Table III).

Table III: Medium-term results

	Total N = 50		Group 1: OS N = 23		Group 2: CS N = 27		p
MACE (%)	7	(14%)	3	(13)	4	(15)	0,11
Mortality (%)	1	(2%)	0		1	(4)	0,3
IDM (%)	2	(4%)	1	(4)	1	(4)	0,87
TLR (%)	4	(8%)	2	(9)	2	(7)	0,67
- RIS	3		1		2		
- TS	1		1		0		

CS: crossover stenting; MI: myocardial infarction; MACE: major adverse cardiac events; OS: ostial stenting; RIS: intrastent restenosis; TLR: target lesion revascularisation; ST: stent thrombosis.

DISCUSSION

1- Main results of our study

We conducted a single-centre, retrospective, descriptive study at the cardiology department of Mongi Slim La Marsa Hospital over a three-year period from January 2019 to December 2021. 50 consecutive patients with significant ostial IVA stenosis, excluding TCG stenosis, were included and divided into two groups according to angioplasty technique (OS group: 23 patients and CS group: 27 patients). The two groups were comparable in terms of demographic and clinical characteristics, with a predominance of males. Smoking (94%) followed by diabetes (62%) and hypertension (40%) were the main risk factors in our population. In terms of angiographic and procedural characteristics, the OS group was distinguished by a shorter stent length, fewer complications at the ostium of the circumflex (Cx) and less use of PDC. Follow-up at one year found no significant difference in terms of MACE and mortality, with low LRT levels in both groups.

2- Strengths and limitations of the study

➢ Highlights of the study

- The relevance of the subject, which always poses a problem for the interventional cardiologist.

- The exhaustive nature of the inclusions means that this work constitutes a real-life study.

➢ Limitations of the study :

- The retrospective and monocentric nature of the study.
- The relatively short inclusion period meant that the number of patients in both groups was limited. This limited the number of MACE and thus the statistical power of the study.

- The angioplasty technique was left to the discretion of the operator.
- Failure to use endocoronary imaging because it is not available.

- Angiographic analysis by a single interventional cardiologist.
- The heterogeneity of the population, including both acute and chronic coronary syndromes.

- The use of bare stents is responsible for a possible increase in MACE.

3- Special features of atheromatous lesions of the ostial IVA :

It has been established that coronary atherosclerosis has an affinity for the ostial and proximal segment of the IVA artery, particularly in its first ten millimetres. This is due to the particular haemodynamic characteristics of the bifurcation of the left common trunk. The ostial VIA undergoes a turbulent, oscillatory arterial flow that is damped by the bifurcation. Combined with endothelial dysfunction, these physical constraints contribute tò atheromatous plaque formation [12-14]. With the development of endocoronary ultrasound, the "in vivo" study of atheromatous plaque has become increasingly important. In a study by Hausmann et al, it was found that in 69% of cases, the atheromatous plaque was located eccentrically in the arterial wall opposite the carina separating the IVA and the circumflex [15].

These proximal lesions have a poorer prognosis than distal

lesions. This hypothesis was put forward by the randomised CASS [16] who demonstrated that, all arteries combined, proximal coronary lesions have a poor prognosis compared with distal lesions.

4- Clinical characteristics of the population

In our series, the mean age of the population was 63.5 ±14 years. In the literature, the average age of patients with isolated ostial AVI lesions is fairly uniform, ranging from 55 to 65 years. The male predominance found in our population (86%) is consistent in all these studies. However, neither age nor male predominance is specific to ostial AVI involvement in coronary artery disease. The rate of diabetes in our study (62%) was significantly higher than in all international studies, where the proportion rarely exceeded 40%, which seems to be a particular feature of the Tunisian population. This high rate of diabetes in the Tunisian population is not only linked to genetic factors, but also to a change in lifestyle (sedentary lifestyle and stress) and the adoption of new eating habits. In our population, the smoking rate was higher than that described in the international literature (around 60%) and even nationally by Abdennadher et al. in 2011 [17].This is linked to the country's precarious socio-economic situation and the failure of anti-smoking strategies. A comparison with the results of the national and international literature is summarised in Table IV.

Table IV: Comparison of the population characteristics of our study with data from the literature

	Year	Number (OS /CS)	Age (OS/CS)	Male (OS /CS) %	Diabetes (OS / CS) %	Tobacco (OS / CS)	CRI (OS / CS)	Stable angina (OS /CS) %
Soylu [18]	2022	97 (56 /	(59.5 ±	(75 /73)	(42,9/	-	-	(44,6/
		41)	13.7		48,8)			53,7)
			61.6±					
			14.7)					
Elkhateeb	2022	175	65 (64,5	77,7	31,4	61,7	-	20
[19]		(150/	/ 67,7)	(78,7/72)	(31,3/32)	(58/84)		(20/20)
		25)						
Rigatelli	2019	74(38	(61,1/	(76,4/	(31,6	-	(31,6 /	0
[20]		/36)	58,9)	72,2)	/50)		44,4)	
BenAyed [21]	2017	76 (46 /30)	59,8±4,4	80	52,6	58,5	12	30
Our	2024	50 (23	63,5	86(87	62(61	94	26	56 (57
study		/27)	(62,7/	/85)	/63)	(91/	(30 /	/55)
			64,1)			96)	22)	

CS: crossover stenting; CKD: chronic renal failure; OS: ostial stenting.

5- Angiographic and procedural particularities

In our study, ostial stenting of the IVA (OS) significantly reduced the length of the stents implanted compared with provisional stenting (CO), as well as complications at the ostium of the Cx with greater use of PDC. This was also noted by Rigatelli et al [20] in 2019.The kissing balloon was not commonly used in our series (only one case in the CS group), as this simplified the procedure apart from significant pinching of the ostium of the Cx. The kissing balloon does not appear to be necessary in single-stent techniques, but is becoming mandatory in the management of double-stent bifurcations. Procedural success was achieved in almost all patients (49), demonstrating a safe and reliable procedure whatever the technique used. This is in line with national and international series [18-21].

6- Medium-term prognosis

In our series, the rate of MACE and mortality at one year were low, with no significant difference between the two angioplasty techniques. This is in agreement with the recent study by Elkhateeb et al [19]. Conversely, two other studies in 2019 [20] and 2022 [18] suggest a reduction in MACE with crossover stenting, but without any significant difference in mortality.

7- What is the best angioplasty technique for isolated de novo lesions of the ostial IVA in the light of contemporary data?

When faced with isolated ostial damage to the LAI, the interventional cardiologist is faced with the dilemma of exclusive ostial stenting or coverage of the left common trunk, with the risk of transforming a single lesion in one vessel into a complex lesion in three vessels. If the stent is incorrectly positioned, ostial stenting may lead to incomplete coverage of the ostium or, conversely, excessive protrusion into the TCG.

For this reason, several techniques have been developed to improve positioning exactly at the ostium of the IVA :

- Stent draw back technique [22]

Described by Schwartz et al. for bifurcation lesions, this technique requires the se of a second guide placed in the collateral branch. The stent is first advanced beyond the lesion on the guide of the target vessel. A compliant balloon is advanced over the second guide then inflated opposite the ostial lesion at low pressure (6-8 atm). The stent is withdrawn until an indentation is seen on the balloon, at which point the stent is released and the two balloons deflated.

- Partial IVA stent pre-inflation technique [23]

Stent deployment in the ostial IVA is often hampered by the oscillatory movements of the heart, which cause the stent to move back and forth. Precise stent deployment can be facilitated by low-pressure (2-4 atm) pre-inflation of the balloon on which the stent is mounted. This will stabilise the stent in the stenosis, while allowing precise adjustment of its location prior to deployment.

- Szabo technique [24]

Two guidewires are advanced, one on the IVA artery and one on the circumflex artery. The stent is then mounted on the IVA guide and hooked to the proximal end of the circumflex guide at the proximal mesh of the stent.

The stent is advanced at the level of the ostial IVA lesion until the guide that hooks the proximal meshes prevents forward movement. Discreet bending of this guide indicates correct positioning.

The stent is inflated at low pressure (6-8 atm) before the guide is withdrawn from the circumflex in order to release the stent at high pressure and achieve good deployment with complete coverage of the ostium. In its recent consensus of 2021 [7], the EBC recommends the use of endocoronary imaging to confirm isolated IVA involvement (without TCG plaque) before considering isolated ostial stenting, as angiography alone underestimates TCG involvement.

To opt for isolated ostial stenting, several conditions must be met:

- Open angle between IVA and Cx
- Perfect visualisation of the start of the Cx
- Absence of damage to the TCG

In these conditions, the use of a stent covering the entire ostium of the IVA while extending by a mesh or two "floating" at the level of the bifurcation of the distal left common trunk seems to give the best results [25]. It is simple, safe and reproducible. Although protrusion of a few stent meshes into the bifurcation of the TCG is frequently observed, it is unrelated to the occurrence of subsequent cardiac events. In other cases, particularly where the distal TCG is involved, crossover stenting followed by POT and possibly kissing balloon is recommended.

CONCLUSIONS

Isolated lesions of the ostial VIA are still a challenge for the interventional cardiologist because of their location just downstream of the TCG and upstream of a large vascular territory. The angioplasty technique remains debated to this day, with some advocating focal ostial stenting and others proposing stenting from the TCG to the IVA. In our work, we carried out a monocentric, retrospective and descriptive study in the cardiology department of the Mongi Slim La Marsa Hospital over a three-year period from January 2019 to December 2021 including all ostial IVA angioplasties. We enrolled 50 consecutive patients divided into two groups according to angioplasty technique: group 1 (OS) = 23 patients and group 2 (CS) = 27 patients. The mean age of the patients was 63.5 ±14 years. The two groups were comparable, with a male predominance (SR =6.14) and a high preponderance of smoking (94%) and diabetes (62%) in both groups. The initial clinical presentation was chronic coronary syndrome in more than half the cases (56%). When the stents implanted in the two groups were compared, there was a significant difference, with smaller stent diameter and length in the OS group. Procedural success was achieved in 49 cases (98%). Pinching of the Cx and secondary stenting of the Cx were statistically more frequent in the CS group (p<0.001). Fluoroscopy time did not differ significantly between procedures, but the amount of iodinated contrast medium (ICP) was significantly higher in the OS group.In our study, ostial IVA angioplasty appears to be a safe procedure with acceptable rates of MACE (14%) and low mortality (2%) at one year follow-up, with no statistical difference between the two groups. Clearly, the debate about the optimal technique for percutaneous revascularisation of ostial AVI lesions is ongoing, and larger-scale prospective studies are needed to clarify this issue.

REFERENCES

1-Louvard Y, Thomas M, Dzavik V, Hildick-Smith D, Galassi AR, Pan M, et al. Classification of coronary artery bifurcation lesions and treatments: time for a consensus! Catheter Cardiovasc Interv. 2008;71(2):175-83.

2-Griffith LS, Platia EV, Angell CS, Grunwald L. Coronary arteriographic and electrocardiographic correlates of sudden cardiac death. Acta Med Scandl. 1978;615:43-50.

3-Koenig W, Schinz A, Hofmann H. Proximal left anterior descending coronary heart disease and complex ventricular arrhythmias. Clin Cardiol. 1983;6(2):79-85.

4-Trappe HJ, Lichtlen PR, Klein H, Wenzlaff P, Hartwig CA. Natural history of single vessel disease. Risk of sudden coronary death in relation to coronary anatomy and arrhythmia profile. Eur Heart J. 1989;10(6):514-24.

5-Grottum P, Svindland A, Walloe L. Localization of atherosclerotic lesions in the bifurcation of the main left coronary artery. Atherosclerosis. 1983;47(1):55-62.

6-Singh M, Gersh BJ, McClelland RL, Ho KKL, Willerson JT,

Penny WF, et al. Clinical and Angiographic Predictors of Restenosis After Percutaneous Coronary Intervention. Insights From the Prevention of Restenosis With Tranilast and Its Outcomes (PRESTO) Trial. 2004;109(22):2727-31.

7- Burzotta F, Lassen JF, Lefèvre T, et al. Percutaneous coronary intervention for bifurcation coronary lesions: the 15(th) consensus document from the European Bifurcation Club. EuroIntervention. 2021;16(16):1307-1317.

8- Rigatelli G, Zuin M, Baracca E, et al. Long-term clinical outcomes of isolated ostial left anterior descending disease treatment: ostial stenting versus left main cross-over stenting. Cardiovasc Revasc Med. 2019;20(12):1058-1062.

9- Thygesen K, Alpert JS, Jaffe AS, Simoons ML, Chaitman BR, White HD, et al. Third universal definition of myocardial infarction. Eur Heart J. 2012;33(20):2551-67.

10- Kip KE, Hollabaugh K, Marroquin OC, Williams DO. The problem with composite end points in cardiovascular studies. the story of major adverse cardiac events and percutaneous coronary intervention. J Am Coll Cardiol. 2008;51(7):701-7.

11-Mauri L, Hsieh W, Massaro JM, Ho KKL, D'Agostino R, Cutlip DE. Stent thrombosis in randomized clinical trials of drug-eluting stents. N Engl J Med. 2007;356(10):1020-9.

12-Brown AJ, Teng Z, Evans PC, Gillard JH, Samady H, Bennett MR. Role of biomechanical forces in the natural history of coronary atherosclerosis. Nat Rev Cardiol. 2016;13(4):210-20.

13-Soulis JV, Giannoglou GD, Chatzizisis YS, Farmakis TM, Giannakoulas GA, Parcharidis GE, et al. Spatial and phasic oscillation of non-Newtonian wall shear stress in human left coronary artery bifurcation: an insight to atherogenesis. Coron Artery Dis. 2006;17(4):351-8.

14-Soulis JV, Farmakis TM, Giannoglou GD, Louridas GE. Wall shear stress in normal left coronary artery tree. J Biomech. 2006;39(4):742-9.

15-Hausmann D, Lundkvist AJ, Friedrich G, Sudhir K, Fitzgerald PJ, Yock PG. Lumen and plaque shape in atherosclerotic coronary arteries assessed by in vivo intracoronary ultrasound. Am J Cardiol. 1994;74(9):857-63.

16-Emond M, Mock MB, Davis KB, Fisher LD, Holmes DR, Jr, Chaitman BR, et al. Long- term survival of medically treated patients in the Coronary Artery Surgery Study (CASS) Registry. Circulation. 1994;90(6):2645-57.

17-Abdennadher MM. Isolated coronary ostial anterior interventricular disease: clinical features and therapeutic strategies (A propos de 80 cas) [Thesis]. Medicine: Sfax; 2011. 122p.

18-Soylu K, Yıldırım U, Nasifov M, Uçar H, Taşbulak Ö, Allahverdiyev S, Göktekin Ö. Evaluation of Long-Term Outcomes of Crossover or Focal Ostial Stenting of Left Anterior Descending Artery Ostial Stenosis. Anatol J Cardiol. 2022 Nov;26(11):827-831.

19-Elkhateeb O, Thambi S, Beydoun H, Bishop H, Quraishi A, Kidwai B, Title L. Long-term outcomes following ostial left anterior descending artery intervention with or without crossover to left-main. Am J Cardiovasc Dis. 2022 Apr 15;12(2):73-80. PMID: 35600287; PMCID: PMC9123417.

20-Rigatelli G, Zuin M, Baracca E, et al. Long-term clinical outcomes of isolated ostial left anterior descending disease treatment: ostial stenting versus left main cross-over stenting.

Cardiovasc Revasc Med. 2019;20(12):1058-1062.

21-Ben Ayed H. Angioplasty of the ostial anterior interventricular artery: Clinical features, therapeutic strategies, medium-term results. [Thesis]. Medicine: Tunis; 2017. 96p.

22-Kini AS, Moreno PR, Steinheimer AM, Prattipati M, Suleman J, Kim MC, et al. Effectiveness of the stent pull-back technique for nonaorto ostial coronary narrowings. Am J Cardiol. 2005;96(8):1123-8.

23-Hildick-Smith DJ, Shapiro LM. Ostial left anterior descending coronary artery stent positioning: partial preinflation prevents stent oscillation and facilitates accurate deployment. J Interv Cardiol. 2001;14(4):439-42.

24-Kern MJ, Ouellette D, Frianeza T. A new technique to anchor stents for exact placement in ostial stenoses: the stent tail wire or Szabo technique. Catheter Cardiovasc Interv. 2006;68(6):901-6.

25- Medina A, Martín P, De Lezo JS, Amador C, de Lezo JS, Pan M, et al. Vulnerable Carina Anatomy and Ostial Lesions in the left Anterior Descending Coronary Artery After Floating-Stent Treatment. Revista Española de Cardiología (English Edition). 2009;62(11):12

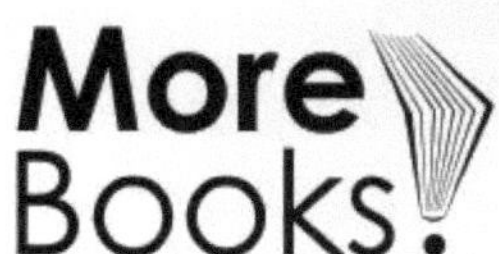

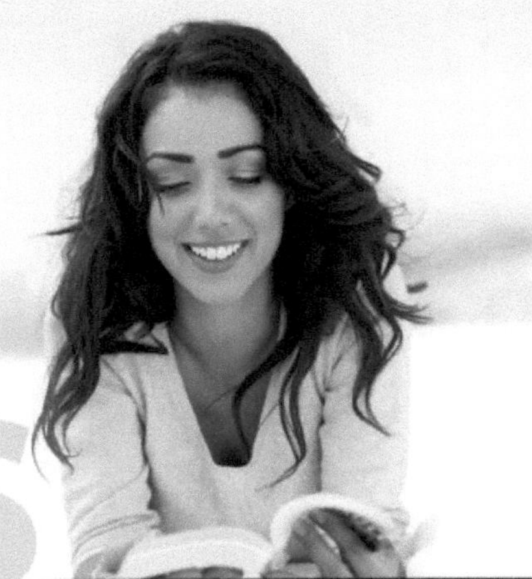

yes

I want morebooks!

Buy your books fast and straightforward online - at one of world's fastest growing online book stores! Environmentally sound due to Print-on-Demand technologies.

Buy your books online at

www.morebooks.shop

Kaufen Sie Ihre Bücher schnell und unkompliziert online – auf einer der am schnellsten wachsenden Buchhandelsplattformen weltweit! Dank Print-On-Demand umwelt- und ressourcenschonend produzi ert.

Bücher schneller online kaufen

www.morebooks.shop

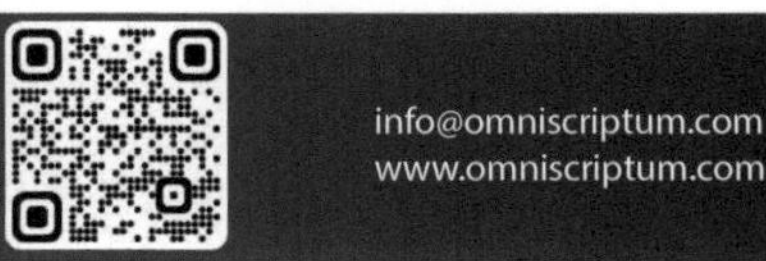

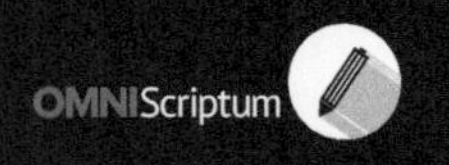

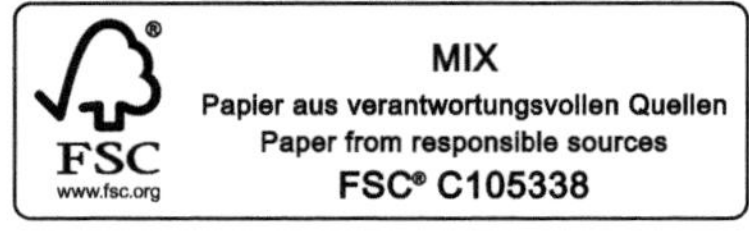

Printed by Books on Demand GmbH, Norderstedt / Germany